THE BEST

5-INGREDIENT KETO

COOKBOOK

Easy and Delicious Ketogenic Diet Recipes For Healthy Living(Low Carb High Fat Recipes) and Keep You On Track (Vol.1)

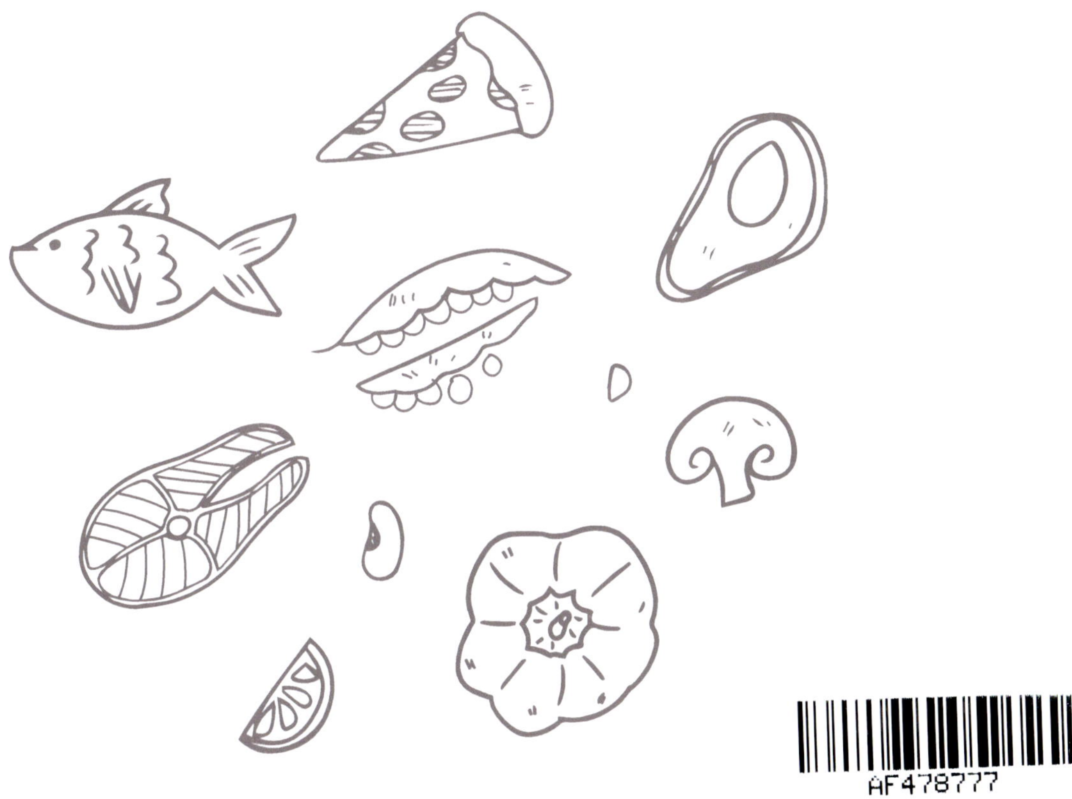

Olvido Mena

CONTENTS

Blue Cheese and Bacon Kale Salad

Chopped Greek Salad

Mediterranean Cucumber Salad

Avocado Egg Salad Lettuce Cups

Avocado Caprese Salad

Shrimp and Avocado Salad

Salmon Caesar Salad

Salmon and Spinach Cobb Salad

Taco Salad

Cheeseburger Salad

California Steak Salad

Skirt Steak Cobb Salad

FOUR Side Dishes & Snacks

Roasted Cauliflower with Prosciutto, Capers, and Almonds

Buttery Slow-Cooker Mushrooms

Baked Zucchini Gratin

Roasted Radishes with Brown Butter Sauce

Parmesan and Pork Rind Green Beans

Pesto Cauliflower Steaks

Tomato, Avocado, and Cucumber Salad

Crunchy Pork Rind and Zucchini Sticks

Cheese Chips and Guacamole

Cauliflower "Potato" Salad

Loaded Cauliflower Mashed "Potatoes,"

Keto Bread

Deviled Eggs

Chicken-Pecan Salad Cucumber Bites

Buffalo Chicken Dip

Roasted Brussels Sprouts with Bacon

Salami, Pepperoncini, and Cream Cheese Pinwheels

Cauliflower Steaks with Bacon and Blue Cheese

Bacon-Wrapped Jalapeños

Creamy Broccoli-Bacon Salad

FIVE Fish & Poultry Entrées

Baked Lemon-Butter Fish

Fish Taco Bowl

Scallops with Creamy Bacon Sauce

Shrimp and Avocado Lettuce Cups

Garlic Butter Shrimp

Parmesan-Garlic Salmon with Asparagus

Seared-Salmon Shirataki Rice Bowls

Pork Rind Salmon Cakes

Creamy Dill Salmon

Chicken-Basil Alfredo with Shirataki Noodles

Chicken Quesadilla

Garlic-Parmesan Chicken Wings

Chicken Skewers with Peanut Sauce

Braised Chicken Thighs with Kalamata Olives

Buttery Garlic Chicken

Cheesy Bacon and Broccoli Chicken

Parmesan Baked Chicken

Crunchy Chicken Milanese

Baked Garlic and Paprika Chicken Legs

Creamy Slow-Cooker Chicken

SIX Pork & Beef Entrées

BLTA Cups

Butter and Herb Pork Chops

Parmesan Pork Chops and Roasted Asparagus

Sesame Pork and Green Beans

Slow-Cooker Barbecue Ribs

Kalua Pork with Cabbage

Pork Burgers with Sriracha Mayo

Blue Cheese Pork Chops

Carnitas

Carnitas Nachos

Pepperoni Low-Carb Tortilla Pizza

Beef and Broccoli Roast

Beef and Bell Pepper "Potato Skins"

Skirt Steak with Chimichurri Sauce

Barbacoa Beef Roast

Steak and Egg Bibimbap

Mississippi Pot Roast

Taco Cheese Cups

Bacon Cheeseburger Casserole

Feta-Stuffed Burgers

SEVEN Desserts & Sweet Treats

Blueberry-Blackberry Ice Pops

Strawberry-Lime Ice Pops

Coffee Ice Pops

Fudge Ice Pops

Root Beer Float

Orange Cream Float

Strawberry Shake

"Frosty" Chocolate Shake

Strawberry Cheesecake Mousse

Lemonade Fat Bomb

Berry Cheesecake Fat Bomb

Peanut Butter Fat Bomb

Crustless Cheesecake Bites

Pumpkin Crustless Cheesecake Bites

Berry-Pecan Mascarpone Bowl

Peanut Butter Cookies

Chocolate Mousse

Mint–Chocolate Chip Ice Cream

Chocolate-Avocado Pudding

Dark-Chocolate Strawberry Bark

EIGHT Sauces & Dressings

Dijon Vinaigrette

Green Goddess Dressing

Caesar Dressing

Avocado-Lime Crema

Chunky Blue Cheese Dressing

Sriracha Mayo

Avocado Mayo

Peanut Sauce

Introduction

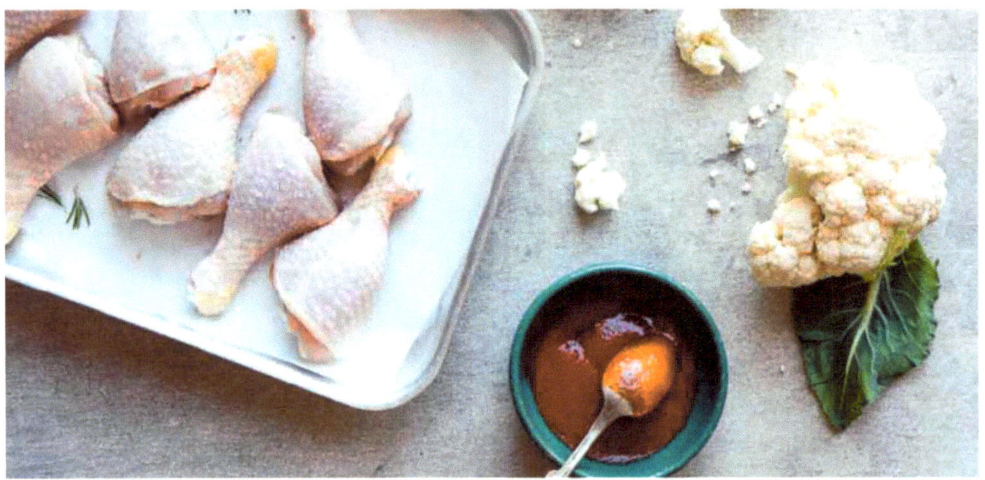

WHAT ON EARTH IS KETOSIS? WHAT IS A MACRO, AND HOW DO I MEASURE IT? I DECIDED TO TRY THE KETO DIET, AND I AM SO GLAD I DID.

I'm so happy you've decided to explore the ketogenic way of eating with me.

Following a keto diet has helped so many people. The keto diet is a super-low-carbohydrate diet that includes a high level of healthy fats and a moderate level of protein. My journey with low-carbohydrate eating began over a decade ago, at the recommendation of a doctor I was seeing for acupuncture. When I was 18 and 19 years old, I was diagnosed with two autoimmune disorders: psoriatic arthritis and psoriasis. I was looking for ways to alleviate pain and inflammation, and the doctor recommended that I cut sugar out of my diet. This was the first time I had thought about the connection between food and autoimmune disorders.

I followed his advice, started on a low-carb diet, cut out sugar, and saw relief within weeks. I noticed a definite decrease in the inflammation in my joints as well as in my skin, which had been angry and red. This started me on a path of discovery, learning more about how my body reacts to various foods and finally finding an eating plan that could help me feel like my best self.

For many years I followed a mostly low-carbohydrate eating plan, but I also went through periods where I "fell off the wagon." Then, a few years ago, I started having more autoimmune issues again. My doctors thought perhaps I had Crohn's disease, but they weren't sure. After many tests and not a lot of answers, I decided to go back to experimenting with food to see if I could help heal myself. I started by eating high-quality foods (organic, grass-fed, etc.) but with gluten-free carbs. I saw some improvement with my issues, but I just felt sluggish, and after six months of following that plan, I had gained weight thanks to those tasty gluten-free treats that are so readily available these days.

Then I came across the ketogenic diet. At first, it seemed like the induction phase to the Atkins diet, but I liked the idea of eating real foods, lower in protein, with a focus on healthy fats. I had never heard of "keto" at the time, and like many people, I felt a little confused and overwhelmed by the new keto terms. What on Earth is ketosis? What is a macro, and how do I measure it? But I decided to try the keto diet, and I am so glad I did.

Immediately I loved the challenge of creating keto-friendly meals that were quick and easy, and also delicious. I am a single mom, and I work full time. I also have an extremely busy teenage daughter, so I like to keep recipes (and everything else in my life) as simple as humanly possible. In my experience, you do not need a lot of exotic ingredients and a cup-board full of special oils to whip up amazing keto meals.

The recipes in this book will help satisfy cravings you will have for those high-carb favorites you used to eat pre-keto. Having those cravings is super normal. Most people have eaten a high-carbohydrate diet their entire lives, so it is definitely an adjustment to go keto. But I encourage you to stick with it.

My 5-ingredient recipes have made my life easier. For this book, I created as many recipes as I could that can be made in 30 minutes or less. Who has the time these days to spend hours preparing a meal? The recipes are full of flavor and healthy fats. You'll be cooking with natural, wholesome ingredients that are easy to find and that are affordable. There is no need to go to five different grocery stores just to hunt down a bunch of unfamiliar ingredients. My recipes make keto easy!

Come along with me as I guide you on your keto journey. I know you can do it. I'm excited to show you all the super-delicious ways you can make my easy, 5-ingredient, keto-friendly recipes. Let's start cooking!

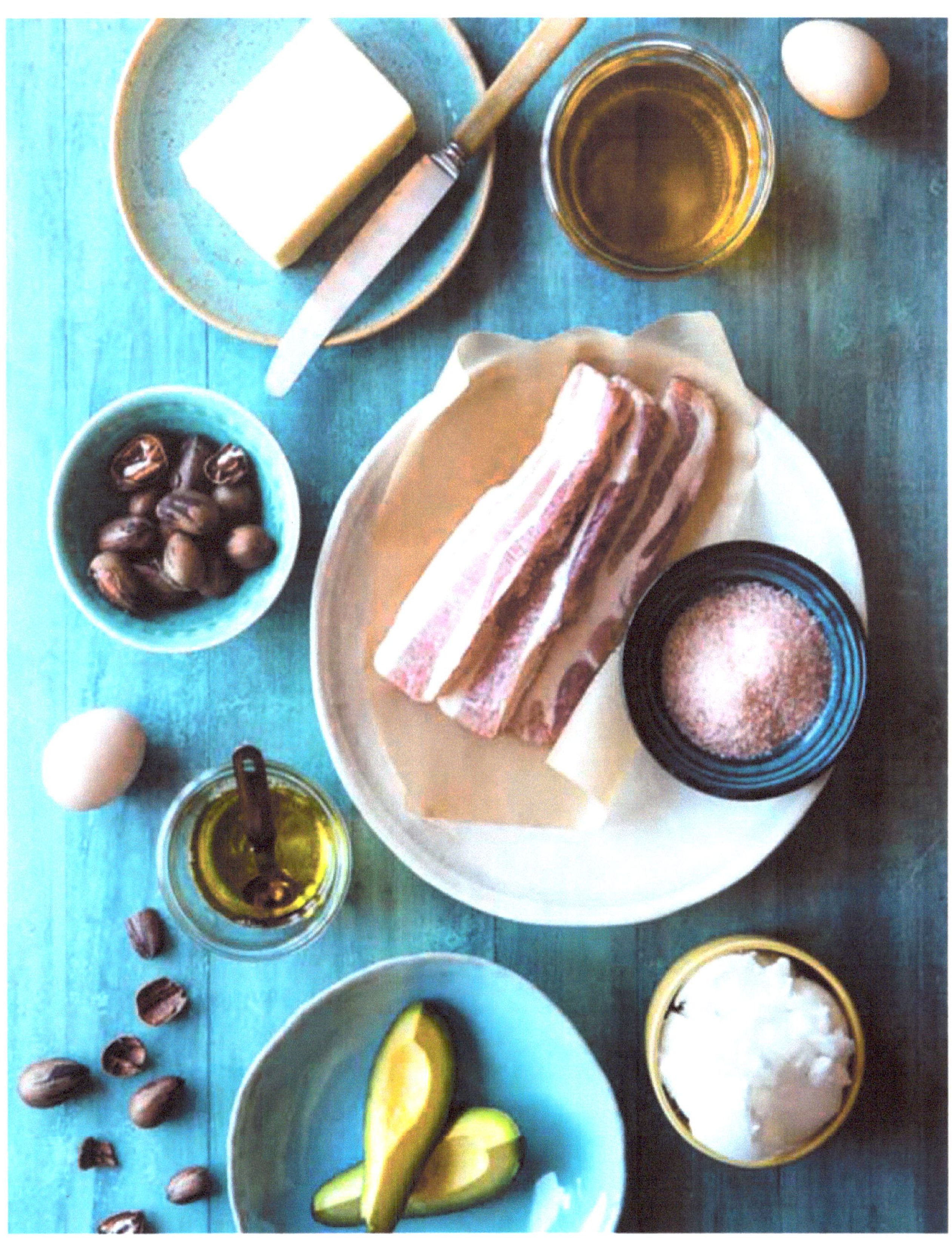

ONE

SIMPLE & EASY KETOGENIC COOKING

What I love most about the ketogenic lifestyle is how easy it is, both when cooking at home and eating out. The recipes in this book are simple and use familiar foods. I will show you how to turn everyday, easy-to-find ingredients into keto-friendly meals that are delicious and full of the healthy fats your body will use to fuel itself. The most important step in starting the keto diet is just starting! Don't feel intimidated: I will walk you through everything you need to know!

HOW THE KETO DIET WORKS

Starting a new eating plan can be overwhelming. I know when I first started researching the ketogenic diet online, the materials available were confusing, and I felt like I was back in science class. But at its core, "keto" is focused on eating a diet full of healthy fats, mixed with proteins and very few carbs. Ideally, the carbs you do eat will come mainly from vegetables. Your body will switch from burning sugar and carbs for energy to burning fat/ketones for energy. This process is called "ketosis," and it puts you in the optimal state for burning body fat and losing weight. But weight loss is not the only benefit to the keto plan. Mental clarity, reduced inflammation, and increased energy are just some of the other benefits.

When you are first beginning the keto diet, you may find yourself eating more to feel full. But quickly, as you become keto-adapted, you will find that you are often not hungry at mealtime. It is important to learn to listen to your body, and if you are not hungry, you don't need to eat. I continuously remind myself of this lesson. When I am at work, I often feel like I need to eat at noon when everyone goes to lunch. However, on the weekends, without such a schedule, I can often go until 2 or 3 p.m. before eating. Allow your body to guide you, but always make sure you are drinking plenty of water and getting the proper intake of electrolytes.

The benefits of a ketogenic diet are vast, and each person has their own reason for embarking on a keto journey. For me, I was focused on reducing inflammation in my body. Removing sugar, which is extremely inflammatory, and carbohydrates has been life changing. Enabling your body to be in nutritional ketosis can be helpful for conditions such as obesity, epilepsy, neurological conditions, and more. Being a fat burner instead of a sugar burner may also boost your longevity. It seems like every week there are new studies supporting the keto lifestyle.

When starting a ketogenic diet, you may encounter new terms and have some questions:

What is ketosis? Drastically restricting carbs and sugar in your diet puts your body into a state of ketosis, which is when the body burns fat (ketones) instead of glucose (carbs and sugar). When there are very few carbohydrates in the diet, the liver converts fat into fatty acids and ketone bodies. The ketone bodies pass into the brain and replace glucose as an energy source. This elevated level of ketone bodies in the blood is known as ketosis. You can often achieve a state of ketosis within the first week of starting a keto diet, which is the first step of eventually becoming keto-adapted, which can often take about a month to achieve.

What are macros, and why are they important? When you first start a keto diet, you will want to calculate your "macros" and track them every day. Macros, or macronutrients, are the major nutritional elements that make up the caloric content of your food—protein, carbohydrates, fat, plus some minerals. The Centers for Disease Control and Prevention states that the typical American diet is about 50 percent carbohydrates, 15 percent protein, and 35 percent fat. In contrast, the structure of a typical keto diet is closer to 5 percent carbs, 20 to 25 percent protein, and 70 to 75 percent fat.

To find the best macros for you, you can go on Google and search for "keto macro calculator." The macro calculator will ask you to enter information (height, weight, activity level, goals, etc.), and based on that information, it will suggest your keto macros. The macros represent the upper limit of your ideal nutritional intake for each day. Macros will be broken down into calories, fat, protein, and carbohydrates. If weight loss is your goal, it is often recommended that you stay under 20 net carbs per day, which is my daily goal. I use the free Carb Manager application to track my food. You can set the preferences to net carbs.

Some people monitor their total carbohydrates while on the keto diet, and some follow net carbs; it is a personal decision. I count net carbs, which basically means that you subtract the insoluble fiber content from the total carbs because fiber is a carbohydrate that your body cannot digest. For example, ½ cup of cauliflower has 2.65 grams of carbohydrates and 1.2 grams of insoluble fiber. So you subtract the fiber from the total carbohydrates, and the net carb content of that serving is 1.45 grams.

Is eating that much fat good for you? Eating 70 to 75 percent fat on the keto diet probably seems a little crazy when you are used to a typical high-carb, low-fat diet. In fact, when I first started on the keto plan, I found it easy to quit carbs but much more difficult to hit my recommended fat amount every day. The most important thing to remember is that you want to eat high-quality fats; not all fats are created equal! High-quality fats like grass-fed butter, ghee (clarified butter), grass-fed meats, organic full-fat dairy, avocados, macadamia nuts, and salmon are examples of the kinds of fats you want to consume. You should avoid low-quality fats like vegetable or canola oils. You will notice that on the keto plan, you won't be hungry as often because the high-quality fats will keep you satisfied and feeling full.

What is intermittent fasting? Intermittent fasting (IF) can be adopted as part of a ketogenic lifestyle. I typically eat all my food for a day within an eight-hour "eating window," which for me is typically between noon and 8 p.m. This leaves 16 hours in the day where I am intermittently fasting, but I am sleeping for a good portion of that, which makes IF pretty easy to achieve. During the IF time period, I drink Bulletproof Coffee which is allowed on the Bulletproof Intermittent Fasting protocol, and water, but I don't consume any solid food. The Bulletproof Coffee curbs my appetite because of the fat content in the grass-fed butter and Brain Octane Oil. The longer you are on the ketogenic diet, the less hungry you will become in general, because the higher amount of fat you are eating will satiate you.

What is keto-adapted? Most people reach a state of ketosis within a couple of weeks of following their ketogenic macros, but becoming keto-adapted takes a little longer. Once keto-adapted, your body has switched over from using glucose as its main source of energy to using fat for energy. This process generally happens within a month of sticking to a ketogenic diet and producing a certain ketone level.

For more in-depth and scientific information on the ketogenic diet, I highly recommend everyone read *The Ketogenic Bible* by Jacob Wilson Ph.D. and Ryan Lowery. It is the most authoritative and thorough explanation of all things keto.

GUIDELINES FOR THE KETOGENIC DIET

Switching your body from glucose burning to fat burning is a big change. And with change comes a period of adjustment. When you first begin a ketogenic diet, it is important to monitor your electrolytes, focus on nutrient-dense foods, and get plenty of rest during this time of healing for your body. Electrolytes are certain nutrients or chemicals in the body that have many important functions, including stimulating muscles, nerves, maintaining cellular function, regulating your heartbeat, and more. If your electrolytes are out of balance, you will feel tired or just "off."

Manage your electrolytes to minimize the "keto flu" when you are first starting keto. When you begin to follow a ketogenic diet, your body will go through a detox period as it flushes out the carbohydrates and sugar in your system. If you are like most people, you have been eating carbs your whole life, so your body will be making a big adjustment. You may experience side effects, such as lightheadedness, muscle cramps, headaches, nausea, and fatigue. Stay strong; this detox period is only temporary. The key to minimizing the side effects is managing your electrolytes in these ways:

- Drink plenty of water with electrolytes. I prefer Smartwater.

- Get plenty of salt. Consume pink Himalayan salt or broth (meat or veggie), or you can even drink shots of pickle juice.

- Eat foods rich in potassium but low in sugar, like avocado and spinach.

- Eat foods rich in magnesium, like nuts, spinach, artichokes, and fish.

- Get plenty of rest, because your body is healing.

Drink a lot of water. Throughout your keto journey, you will need to drink a lot of water, likely more than you are currently drinking. In the beginning stages of the diet, you will be shedding a lot of water. The carbs in your body tend to hold on to water, and when you stop eating them, your body will begin to release that water, so you need to replenish it. A good guide is to make sure you get *at least* half your body weight in ounces of water daily. For example, if you weigh 200 pounds, you should drink at least 100 ounces of water (a bit more than 3 quarts) every day.

Get plenty of salt. In a standard American diet, people are typically eating foods that have a lot of salt added to them: bread, for example. On keto you are not, so don't be afraid to salt your food (using high-quality salt), and if you feel like you still need more salt, sip some meat or vegetable broth. I recommend pink Himalayan salt because it has more minerals than traditional table salt, such as potassium, magnesium, copper, and iron.

Find easy ways to get your fat in. It may sound daunting to consume 70 to 75 percent of your daily diet in fat, but there are lots of easy ways to take it in throughout the day.

The easiest way is to add butter and/or healthy oils to almost everything you eat.

Do your research before eating out. One of the things I really love about the keto diet is that I can find something keto-friendly on almost any restaurant menu, but it does take some practice! If you can, before you go out, look online at the restaurant's menu to figure out the good keto options. Meat and vegetables are usually a great place to start. Be careful with sauces, dressings, and marinades; they can have lots of hidden carbohydrates. When in doubt, ask your server for the ingredients in the sauces, and if they don't know, I suggest asking to have the sauce left off. Restaurants are used to special requests, so don't be afraid to ask for exactly what you do and don't want.

Ketogenic or Paleo?

KETO AND PALEO ARE TWO DIFFERENT EATING PLANS, BUT THE TERMS OFTEN GET USED INTERCHANGEABLY.

A TYPICAL PALEO DIET is not as high in fat or as low in carbs as the keto diet is. Paleo is all about eating like people did several thousand years ago, when there were no processed foods and they consumed foods they could hunt, like meats, and gather, like nuts, seeds, and plants. On a Paleo diet you can eat sweet potatoes and other high-carbohydrate vegetables like carrots. There are many types of Paleo diets, but on a standard Paleo diet, the macros tend to be closer to 20 percent carbs, 15 percent protein, and 65 percent fat.

ON THE KETO DIET, you shouldn't eat those high-carb vegetables and starches because they will raise your glucose levels and kick you out of ketosis. Keto macros are 5 percent carbs, 20 percent protein, and 75 percent fat. To successfully follow a ketogenic diet, your body must be in a state of ketosis; otherwise, you are simply following a low-carb eating plan.

DAIRY IS ANOTHER DIFFERENTIATOR. On keto, full-fat dairy can be a great way to help you get your healthy fats, but you don't have to eat dairy. In the most traditional form of Paleo diet, dairy is avoided completely, but now there are many types of Paleo plans, and some do allow dairy products.

IT IS POSSIBLE TO FOLLOW THE KETO DIET WHILE ALSO FOLLOWING SOME PALEO PRINCIPLES, particularly a focus on natural, high-quality foods. I always recommend that whenever you can, you use the highest-quality ingredients you can afford. In addition, you can swap out certain ingredients for more Paleo-friendly ingredients; for example, you can replace butter with ghee, and heavy whipping cream with coconut milk.

KITCHEN EQUIPMENT

You don't need to have a bunch of fancy equipment in your kitchen to cook the recipes in this book. But you should have a few key items for everyday use.

MUST HAVE

Measuring cups and measuring spoons You will want to make sure you are measuring items accurately rather than just eyeballing them, especially for the baking recipes. And if weight loss is your goal, portion sizes will be important, too.

Spatula, slotted spoon, large spoon, whisk, tongs, and rubber scraper I tend to buy cute rubber scrapers all the time, but you really only need one of each of these six tools.

Cutting board Ideally you should have two: one for vegetables and one for meat.

Knives Buy one or two quality chef's knives. A quality paring knife and a 6-inch chef's knife are a good start. I bought mine on sale at Williams-Sonoma.

Cheese grater/zester It is less expensive to grate your own cheese than to buy it preshredded. Some graters even have storage containers attached to them for convenience. A citrus zester can also be handy if you find a cheese grater to be too large. In a few of these recipes, we'll also be zesting/shredding citrus and vegetables.

Baking sheet You will want to have one large baking sheet for one-pan meals and for baking.

9-by-13-inch baking pan I like to use a deeper baking pan for roasting vegetables and meat. I also use it for my egg frittatas. The one I use all the time is an easy-to-clean Le Creuset enameled cast iron pan.

9-by-5-inch loaf pan This is a standard-size loaf pan that I use for baking my Keto Bread.

Muffin tin You'll need a standard muffin tin for several of these recipes. I use a jumbo muffin tin for my BLTA Cups, but a standard tin will work here, too.

8-inch glass baking dish A smaller deep glass pan is great for baking desserts or making foods in smaller portions.

10- or 12-inch skillet I like to use a nonstick skillet because they are easy to clean and work really well for keto staples like eggs. Professional chefs would say a nonstick pan won't achieve the same level of sear as a stainless skillet, but for my purposes it works just fine. If you prefer a stainless skillet, you will just need to put a bit more elbow grease into the cleaning process. Whichever you choose, buy one with a lid.

Saucepans Having a small (2-quart) and a large (4.5-quart) saucepan will allow you to make most recipes.

Slow cooker A slow cooker, like the original Crock-Pot and other brands, is very handy for making easy one-dish meals, especially in the winter. I love letting my house fill up with delicious aromas as the food cooks all day long. The cooker I have is super simple—it doesn't have a timer or any other fancy mechanisms—and it works like a dream. I use a 6-quart slow cooker for all the slow cooker recipes in this book.

Colander A colander is important for washing fresh fruits and vegetables. Just a medium-size colander should be adequate unless you are cooking for a crowd.

Mixing bowls A set of nesting mixing bowls is very helpful when making a recipe. I have a set that I have had for at least 10 years, and I use the pieces all the time.

Ice pop molds There are a lot of fun ice pop molds out there, and you can choose any shape to make delicious keto-friendly ice pops.

Parchment paper I use parchment paper for everything from egg frittatas to roasting vegetables to making cheese chips. I buy the precut squares. It says on the box that parchment paper can be used for temperatures up to 425°F. (I learned the hard way!)

You will also need either a blender or a food processor:

Blender A blender is a great tool for making smoothies, coffee drinks, soups, and sauces. If you don't have a blender, you can get away with doing what I do, which is use my food processor for everything!

Food processor I use my food processor a lot for making these recipes. I have a small one, the Cuisinart Mini-Prep, because there are only two people in my household. It costs about $40, and I use it all the time.

NICE TO HAVE

Mixer I use an electric hand mixer I've had for years, but if you have a countertop mixer, that is an awesome tool. A mixer is particularly helpful for making desserts. If you don't have either, you can also use a whisk and get a great arm workout at the same time.

Kitchen scale I do not have a kitchen scale, but I know it is a key item for many people who are trying to lose weight on keto. They use it to measure portions, especially for meat and other proteins.

Immersion blender This tool is very handy for quickly blending soups and sauces right in the pan or bowl, instead of in a food processor or countertop blender.

Rolling pin If you have a rolling pin, it will come in handy for making dishes like pinwheels. If you don't have one, I have also used a wine bottle and it worked just fine!

Basting brush I like using a basting brush with olive oil so that you don't dump too much, but if you don't have one, you can also use a leafy green or paper towel instead.

Cooling rack For several of these recipes, I transfer a finished dish from the oven to a cooling rack. If you don't have one, setting your hot dishes on trivets or pot holders will work, too.

FOODS TO ENJOY

HIGH FAT / LOW CARB (BASED ON NET CARBS)

MEATS & SEAFOOD

Beef (ground beef, steak, etc.)

Chicken

Crab

Crawfish

Duck

Fish

Goose

Lamb

Lobster

Mussels

Octopus

Pork (pork chops, bacon, etc.)

Quail

Sausage (without fillers)

Scallops

Shrimp

Veal

Venison

DAIRY

Blue cheese dressing

Burrata cheese

Cottage cheese

Cream cheese

Eggs

Greek yogurt (full-fat)

Grilling cheese

Halloumi cheese

Heavy (whipping) cream

Homemade whipped cream

Kefalotyri cheese

Mozzarella cheese

Provolone cheese

Queso blanco

Ranch dressing

Ricotta cheese

Unsweetened almond milk

Unsweetened coconut milk

NUTS & SEEDS

Almonds

Brazil nuts

Chia seeds

Flaxseeds

Hazelnuts

Macadamia nuts

Peanuts (in moderation)

Pecans

Pine nuts

Pumpkin seeds

Sacha inchi seeds

Sesame seeds

Walnuts

FRUITS & VEGETABLES

Alfalfa sprouts

Asparagus

Avocados

Bell peppers

Blackberries

Blueberries

Broccoli

Cabbage

Carrots (in moderation)

Cauliflower

Celery

Chicory

Coconut

Cranberries

Cucumbers

Garlic (in moderation)

Green beans

Herbs

Jicama

Lemons

Limes

Mushrooms

Okra

Olives

Onions (in moderation)

Pickles

Pumpkin

Radishes

Raspberries

Salad greens

Scallions

Spaghetti squash (in moderation)

Strawberries

Tomatoes (in moderation)

Zucchini

FOODS TO AVOID

LOW FAT / HIGH CARB (BASED ON NET CARBS)

MEATS & MEAT ALTERNATIVES

Deli meat (some, not all)

Hot dogs (with fillers)

Sausage (with fillers)

Seitan

Tofu

DAIRY

Almond milk (sweetened)

Coconut milk (sweetened)

Milk

Soy milk (regular)

Yogurt (regular)

NUTS & SEEDS

Cashews

Chestnuts

Pistachios

FRUITS & VEGETABLES

Apples

Apricots

Artichokes

Bananas

Beans (all varieties)

Boysenberries

Burdock root

Butternut squash

Cantaloupe

Cherries

Chickpeas

Corn

Currants

Dates

Edamame

Eggplant

Elderberries

Gooseberries

Grapes

Honeydew melon

Huckleberries

Kiwifruits

Leeks

Mangos

Oranges

Parsnips

Peaches

Peas

Pineapples

Plantains

Plums

Potatoes

Prunes

Raisins

Sweet potatoes

Taro root

Turnips

Water chestnuts

Winter squash

Yams

KETO PANTRY ESSENTIALS

It is wise to have a well-stocked pantry when you are cooking keto meals. You do not need any exotic cooking ingredients; you just need to have the basics. Each recipe in this book has only 5 main ingredients, but the following 5 basic cooking staples do *not* count toward those ingredients.

KETO COOKING STAPLES

1. Pink Himalayan salt

2. Freshly ground black pepper

3. Ghee (clarified butter, without dairy; buy grass-fed if you can)

4. Olive oil

5. Grass-fed butter

In addition to these 5 staples, there are 10 key perishable ingredients you will want to always have on hand. I recommend that you purchase organic/all-natural whenever possible.

KETO PERISHABLES

1. Eggs (pasture-raised, if you can)

2. Avocados

3. Bacon (uncured)

4. Cream cheese (full-fat; or use a dairy-free alternative)

5. Sour cream (full-fat; or use a dairy-free alternative)

6. Heavy whipping cream or coconut milk (full-fat; I buy the coconut milk in a can)

7. Garlic (fresh or pre-minced in a jar)

8. Cauliflower

9. Meat (grass-fed, if you can)

10. Greens (spinach, kale, or arugula)

In addition, the following are some of my favorite products that I always keep in my kitchen. Some are staples and some are snacks or sweet treats. In the Resources section, I tell you where to find these products. I even have discount codes you can use for some of them!

FAVORITE KETO PRODUCTS

Vital Farms Pasture-Raised Eggs The first thing that attracted me to this brand of eggs was their beautiful packaging and the fact that these eggs are pasture raised. The yolks are orange, and the eggs are delicious; buying pasture-raised eggs definitely makes a difference. Fresh pasture-raised eggs are even better if you have a local farmers' market.

Kerrygold Butter Grass-fed butter just tastes better; once you switch, you will never go back. Kerrygold, from Ireland, has a higher fat content. There are other grass-fed brands, but Kerrygold is widely available at Whole Foods, Costco, Trader Joe's, Walmart, and Safeway. It comes unsalted and salted; I use salted for almost everything.

Bulletproof Brain Octane Oil Bulletproof is a brand that makes a variety of high-quality keto products. My favorites

are their coffee, ghee, and Brain Octane Oil. The Brain
Octane Oil is one of my keto secret weapons because it is a
very easy way to add high-quality fats to anything you eat.
One tablespoon of the oil has 14 grams of fat, no flavor, and
no smell. I use Brain Octane Oil in my Bulletproof Coffee,
often called "butter coffee," and there are many other ways
to use it.

Bulletproof Ghee I trust the quality of Bulletproof
products, so I also purchase their ghee. Ghee is clarified
butter (with no dairy), which has a high smoke point, so it is
great to use for cooking. Just like with butter, I recommend
grass-fed ghee. A good percentage of people who do the keto
diet do it dairy-free, so ghee is a perfect replacement for
butter in cooking, as well as a tasty addition to Bulletproof
Coffee.

Primal Palate Spice Mixes Seasoning can really enhance
a dish and a meal. I have fallen in love with the seasoning
mixes from Primal Palate. Their spices are the highest
quality available, and they make amazing spice blends, like
Breakfast Blend, Super Gyro, and Garam Masala, which will
take your dishes to a new level.

Perfect Keto MCT Oil Powder This product is wonderful
for adding high-quality fats in dishes and drinks. Oils can be
messy and of course add an oily texture to drinks. MCT oil
powder adds fats, and it has a nice creamy texture that
works perfectly in beverages like coffee or smoothies. I also
use it in baking because it doesn't have a taste, and it just
adds healthy fats.

Perfect Keto Protein Collagen MCT Oil Powder Also by
Perfect Keto, this dairy-free protein powder has collagen in

it, which I love. The production of collagen in our bodies slows down as we age, so consuming products like this one with added collagen can help combat some of the collagen loss. Collagen is beneficial for the joints, hair, and nails, among other things.

Fat Snax Cookies These healthy, fat-packed cookies come in delicious flavors and are Paleo-friendly, keto-friendly, and organic. My daughter loves to make keto-friendly ice cream sandwiches with them.

Keto Kookies Another sweet cookie option, Keto Kookie was created by two friends who lost weight on a ketogenic diet and decided to launch their own brand. They come in delicious flavors, and the texture is moist and chewy.

Trader Joe's Rosemary Marcona Almonds I am obsessed with these nuts. If you have never had a Marcona almond, they are an oilier almond with a flatter shape and a delicate taste. Trader Joe's sells a couple of varieties, but rosemary is my favorite.

Miracle Noodles and Miracle Rice These two products really expand what you can do with keto cooking. Miracle Noodles and Miracle Rice are gluten-free, soy-free, and calorie-free and have zero net carbs. They have a variety of noodle styles so you can make all your favorite noodle dishes in a keto-friendly way.

Primal Kitchen Products For mayo and salad dressings, I love Primal Kitchen's products. If you aren't going to make your own, this is the brand I would trust. Their mayo is made with avocado oil and is sugar-free.

I'm also fond of using the following general, non-keto-specific products for my recipes. They taste great, fulfill my dietary requirements, and tend to be reasonably priced. All of my recipes were tested and developed using these products, but feel free to substitute alternatives if you have your own favorites!

- Annie's Organic Honey Mustard Dressing

- Boar's Head or Citterio Pancetta

- Bob's Red Mill Coconut Flour

- Elvio's Chimichurri Sauce

- Frank's RedHot Sauce

- Justin's All Natural Peanut Butter

- Kettle & Fire Bone Broth

- Lily's Sugar-Free Chocolate Chips

- Mission Low-Carb Whole-Wheat Tortillas

- Muir Glen Organic Diced Tomatoes with Italian Seasoning

- Organic Girl Fresh Salad Greens: Baby Spinach, Baby Kale, Romaine Hearts, Romaine Leaves, Butter Lettuce, Red Romaine, Baby Arugula

- Primal Kitchen sauces and salad dressings: Mayonnaise, Greek Vinaigrette, Caesar with Avocado Oil, Ranch

- Rao's Homemade Tomato Sauce

- Spicy Red Pepper Miso Mayo

- Swerve Natural Sweetener

- Trader Joe's Almond Flour

- Trader Joe's Chunky Blue Cheese Dressing

- Trader Joe's Coconut Oil Cooking Spray

- Trader Joe's Frozen Medium Cooked Shrimp

- Trader Joe's Organic Chia Seeds

- Trader Joe's Organic Coconut Cream

- Trader Joe's Organic Full-Fat Unsweetened Coconut Milk (13.5-ounce can); it tends to separate, so stir after opening and before measuring

- Trader Joe's Sliced Prosciutto

- Wild Planet Alaska Wild Canned Salmon

- Zevia All-Natural Root Beer

KETO COOKING

The ketogenic diet can seem complicated at first, but it is really about simplifying your eating habits. I am successful when I eat simple meals made with high-quality, natural ingredients. The recipes in this book are good examples of this simple approach, because they each have just 5 main ingredients. By planning your shopping trips around these recipes, you will be able to set yourself up for success. In my experience, the better your plan, the more successful you will be on your keto diet. A "plan" can be different for everyone. For example, I always pack keto-friendly snacks when I go out of town and when I have all-day meetings. Otherwise, it is easy to give in to what is available. For others, preparing an entire week's worth of food on the weekend may be the best plan for success.

Use the highest-quality ingredients you can afford. Processed and lower-quality foods can cause inflammation in your body, which is what a ketogenic diet is fighting against. So do what you can to keep your diet as clean as possible with real, high-quality foods.

Remove non-keto foods from your home. Give away your carb-filled pantry items to your friends, neighbors, coworkers, or a charity. Just get them out of the house to set yourself up for success.

Keep your food as simple as possible. Stick to recipes like the ones in this book that use real food and do not have lots of ingredients. Keto is made to be simple.

Track your food throughout the day. Get in the habit of entering your meals into an app like Carb Manager. Not every meal has to add up to perfect keto macros, but the more mindful you are throughout the day, the easier it will be to reach your goals. The macro goals you are aiming for every day are in fat, protein, carbs, and calories.

Plan your meals. Prepping meals ahead of time so you always have food on hand is the key to success for many people. Make sure your refrigerator and pantry are stocked with staples so that when those cravings hit, you can satisfy them with an appropriate low-carb, high-fat option.

Prep and store ingredients ahead of time. Hardboiled eggs make perfect last-minute snacks that you can prepare ahead of time and have ready in the refrigerator. I also like to prepare small zip-top bags of veggies, nuts, slices of cheese, and other keto-friendly snacks, and keep them available in the fridge for grab and go. Also, you will find that rinsing and cutting up vegetables you plan to use for the next week's recipes is a helpful way to cut down on your evening meal-prep time.

Cook in bulk. It is usually cheaper to buy meat and poultry in larger quantities, so don't be reluctant to cook a week's worth at one time and store it in the refrigerator and freezer. It will save you a lot of time throughout the week.

Don't be afraid of new food combinations. The ketogenic diet gives you the opportunity to get creative with delicious high-fat ingredients you may not be very familiar with.

Don't be afraid of salt and seasoning. You can give a dish as simple as eggs a totally different taste profile simply by using different seasonings. Have fun with flavors.

Commit. It takes about a month to become fully keto-adapted, which is when your body has fully switched over and has become super-efficient at using fat/ketones as fuel. Keto is meant to be a long-term way of eating, so give your body time to heal and adjust.

About the Recipes

IN THIS BOOK YOU WILL FIND 130 EASY, 5-INGREDIENT RECIPES FOR EVERY MEAL.

Over half the recipes take less than 30 minutes to prepare, and whenever possible I tried to minimize the pots and pans needed because I love for cleanup to be easy, too.

The recipes in this book have helpful labels you can look for:

ONE POT These recipes can be made in a single pot or bowl.

ONE PAN These recipes can be made in a single skillet, baking dish, or other cooking vessel.

30-MINUTE These recipes will take 30 minutes or less for prep and cooking.

NO COOK These recipes do not involve any cooking.

VEGETARIAN These recipes do not contain any meat.

Each recipe in the book calls for just 5 main ingredients and uses some of the 5 pantry ingredients as well: pink Himalayan salt, freshly ground black pepper, grass-fed ghee, olive oil, and grass-fed butter. You'll find the nutritional information as well as the macro breakdowns (see here) at the bottom of each recipe.

Every recipe also includes at least one tip:

SUBSTITUTION TIP This tip makes suggestions for replacing or swapping out ingredients.

INGREDIENT TIP This tip recommends easy or alternative ways of prepping ingredients.

VARIATIONS This tip suggests other flavor or ingredient combinations you can use in the basic dish to easily change a recipe.

Most of the recipes in the book are made for two people, because I originally created my recipes for me and my daughter. And through my followers, I've discovered that a two-person recipe yield is very popular. If you're expecting more people, just multiply the ingredients.

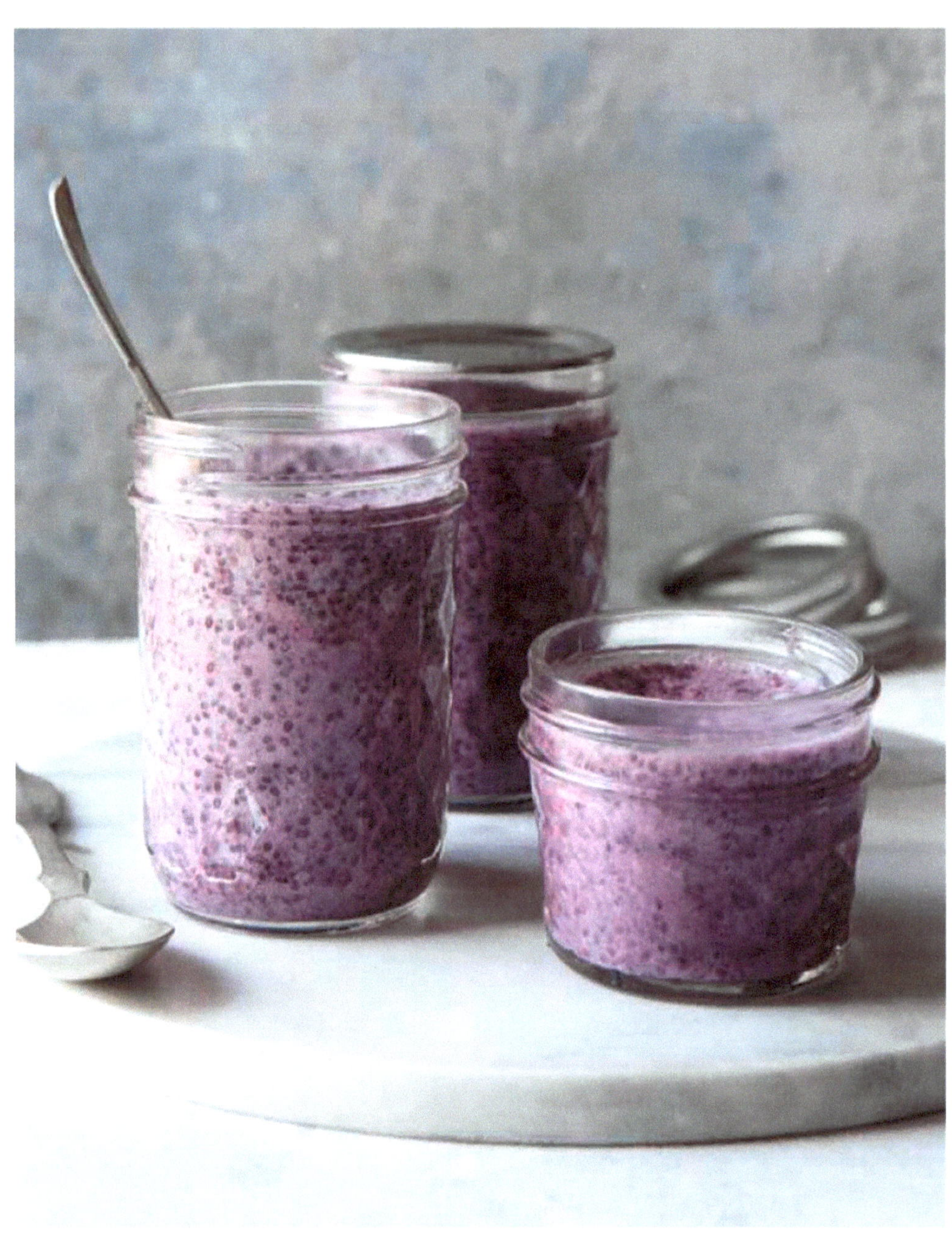

Blackberry-Chia Pudding

SMOOTHIES & BREAKFASTS

The ketogenic diet and breakfast foods are a perfect pair. For just one ingredient, eggs, there are endless ways you can get creative. The recipes in this chapter are some of the favorites I often make for my daughter and me. During the busy work and school week, I generally stick to Bulletproof Coffee or an Americano with heavy whipping cream for breakfast. But on the weekends, I love to make large keto breakfasts. These breakfast recipes will show you how you can take some of your favorite morning dishes, such as sugar- and carb-filled smoothies and pancakes, and turn them into easy, keto-friendly options.

Bulletproof Coffee

Berry-Avocado Smoothie

Almond-Butter Smoothie

Blackberry-Chia Pudding

Double-Pork Frittata

Sausage Breakfast Stacks

Spicy Breakfast Scramble

Bacon-Jalapeño Egg Cups

Bacon and Egg Cauliflower Hash

Bacon, Spinach, and Avocado Egg Wrap

Smoked Salmon and Cream Cheese Roll-Ups

Brussels Sprouts, Bacon, and Eggs

BLT Breakfast Salad

Cheesy Egg and Spinach Nest

Kale-Avocado Egg Skillet

Egg-in-a-Hole Breakfast Burger

Cream Cheese and Coconut Flour Pancakes or Waffles

Pancake "Cake"

Breakfast Quesadilla

Cream Cheese Muffins

BULLETPROOF COFFEE

Bulletproof Coffee is a staple beverage in a lot of keto diets. I love it and honestly feel like Wonder Woman after I drink a cup. One of the biggest benefits for me is being able to extend my Bulletproof intermittent fast because the fat-filled coffee keeps me satiated until lunchtime. If you are not using Bulletproof Coffee for fasting and instead would like to add protein or collagen, you can do that as well.

30-MINUTE

ONE PAN

NO COOK

SERVES 1

PREP 5 minutes

1½ cups hot coffee

2 tablespoons MCT oil powder or Bulletproof Brain Octane Oil

2 tablespoons butter or ghee

1. Pour the hot coffee into the blender.

2. Add the oil powder and butter, and blend until thoroughly mixed and frothy.

3. Pour into a large mug and enjoy.

VARIATIONS

If you want to add protein to your Bulletproof Coffee, here are a couple of suggestions. If you are intermittent fasting, you don't want to add protein because it will end your fast. If you aren't fasting, then try these easy ways to create a more filling breakfast drink:

- Raw egg: To add protein, replace the MCT oil powder with 1 raw egg. Sounds weird, I know, but the egg adds an appealing creamy texture, and although the hot coffee cooks the egg, I promise there will be no hint of cooked proteins.

- Protein and collagen powder: You could also add a scoop or two of protein powder. I like Perfect Keto Collagen, which has a great chocolate flavor that is especially tasty in coffee. The Keto Collagen Powder contains grass-fed collagen, MCT oil powder, and protein powder. The collagen is a good anti-inflammatory addition.

- Spiced: Add 1 teaspoon of cinnamon and a little sweetener to your Bulletproof mixture for a delicious spiced version.

INGREDIENT TIP If you're new to the keto diet, you will want to start slow with the Brain Octane Oil. It is powerful, so you'll want to work your way up to 2 tablespoons over the course of a few weeks.

Per Serving

Calories: 463; Total Fat: 51g; Carbs: 0g; Net Carbs: 0g; Fiber: 0g; Protein: 1g

BERRY-AVOCADO SMOOTHIE

This smoothie is my favorite. It's so delicious, and it's filled with healthy fat, potassium, magnesium, and fiber. Use the liquid stevia if you prefer sweeter smoothies.

SERVES 2

PREP 5 minutes

1 cup unsweetened full-fat coconut milk

1 scoop Perfect Keto Exogenous Ketone Powder in peaches and cream

½ avocado

1 cup fresh spinach

½ cup berries, fresh or frozen (no sugar added if frozen)

½ cup ice cubes

¼ teaspoon liquid stevia (optional)

1. In a blender, combine the coconut milk, protein powder, avocado, spinach, berries, ice, and stevia (if using).

2. Blend until thoroughly mixed and frothy.

3. Pour into a very tall glass and enjoy.

INGREDIENT TIP Adding avocado to a smoothie recipe may sound unusual, but it adds nutrition and healthy fat and contributes a creamy smoothness.

Per Batch

Calories: 709; Total Fat: 68g; Carbs: 27g; Net Carbs: 14g; Fiber: 12g; Protein: 8g

Per Serving

Calories: 355; Total Fat: 40g; Carbs: 16g; Net Carbs: 8g; Fiber: 6g; Protein: 4g

ALMOND BUTTER SMOOTHIE

My daughter feels like she is drinking a milkshake when I make this smoothie for her, but it is very healthy. I love knowing that I can give her something delicious that is also powering her body and mind for hours and hours. Add the liquid stevia, a natural sweetener, if you prefer sweeter smoothies.

30-MINUTE
ONE PAN
NO COOK
VEGETARIAN

SERVES 2

PREP 5 minutes

1 cup unsweetened full-fat coconut milk

1 scoop Perfect Keto Exogenous Ketone Powder in chocolate sea salt

½ avocado

2 tablespoons almond butter

½ cup berries, fresh or frozen (no sugar added if frozen)

½ cup ice cubes

¼ teaspoon liquid stevia (optional)

1. In a blender, combine the coconut milk, protein powder, avocado, almond butter, berries, ice, and stevia (if using).

2. Blend until thoroughly mixed and frothy.

3. Pour into a very tall glass and enjoy.

INGREDIENT TIP You can add 1 teaspoon of turmeric powder to boost this smoothie's anti-inflammatory power. Or you can add 1 tablespoon of chia seeds that have been soaked in coconut milk for at least 20 minutes. The seeds will add extra fiber, iron, calcium, and omega-3 fatty acids to the smoothie.

Per Batch

Calories: 892; Total Fat: 85g; Carbs: 31g; Net Carbs: 17g; Fiber: 14g; Protein: 14g

Per Serving

Calories: 446; Total Fat: 43g; Carbs: 16g; Net Carbs: 9g; Fiber: 7g; Protein: 7g

BLACKBERRY-CHIA PUDDING

I developed this recipe one day when I had a can of coconut milk in my pantry and wanted to find a new way to use it. I reached out to my lovely Instagram followers, and someone suggested I make chia pudding. I whipped up the pudding using blackberries, which are a great low-carb option and they add a lot of great flavor and texture. This sweet treat could be a dessert, but I also enjoy it as a super-delicious breakfast. Loaded with fiber, iron, calcium, and omega-3 fatty acids, chia seeds are one of the most nutritious foods on the planet. It's puzzling that such a tiny food can have so many health benefits, right? The chia seeds soak in the coconut milk and soften overnight to help set the pudding mixture. Chia seeds help slow digestion, and the fat content of this dish helps keep you feeling satisfied for hours.

ONE PAN
NO COOK
VEGETARIAN

SERVES 2

PREP 10 minutes, plus overnight to set

1 cup unsweetened full-fat coconut milk

1 teaspoon liquid stevia 1 teaspoon vanilla extract

½ cup blackberries, fresh or frozen (no sugar added if frozen)

¼ cup chia seeds

1. In a food processor (or blender), process the coconut milk, stevia, and vanilla until the mixture starts to thicken.

2. Add the blackberries, and process until thoroughly mixed and purple. Fold in the chia seeds.

3. Divide the mixture between two small cups with lids, and refrigerate overnight or up to 3 days before serving.

COOKING TIP The first time I made this recipe, I tried whisking the mixture by hand in a bowl instead of using a food processor or blender, assuming it would thicken overnight, but it did not. So using a food processor or blender is a must.

Per Batch

Calories: 873; Total Fat: 75g; Carbs: 46g; Net Carbs: 15g; Fiber: 30g; Protein: 15g

Per Serving

Calories: 437; Total Fat: 38g; Carbs: 23g; Net Carbs: 8g; Fiber: 15g; Protein: 8g

DOUBLE-PORK FRITTATA

I love a frittata. I used to always make them with cheese, but one day I was out of cheese and decided to just add heavy whipping cream. The recipe ended up so fluffy and delicious that I have never gone back. For this recipe, I use all-natural pork lard, available from Fatworks as well as most butchers, or you can use the lard from bacon.

30-MINUTE

SERVES 4

PREP 5 minutes

COOK 25 minutes

1 tablespoon butter or pork lard

8 large eggs

1 cup heavy (whipping) cream

Pink salt

Freshly ground black pepper

4 ounces pancetta, chopped

2 ounces prosciutto, thinly sliced

1 tablespoon chopped fresh dill

1. Preheat the oven to 375°F. Coat a 9-by-13-inch baking pan with the butter.

2. In a large bowl, whisk the eggs and cream together. Season with pink salt and pepper, and whisk to blend.

3. Pour the egg mixture into the prepared pan. Sprinkle the pancetta in and distribute evenly throughout.

4. Tear off pieces of the prosciutto and place on top, then sprinkle with the dill.

5. Bake for about 25 minutes, or until the edges are golden and the eggs are just set.

6. Transfer to a rack to cool for 5 minutes.

7. Cut into 4 portions and serve hot.

VARIATIONS

The great part about a frittata is that you can add so many other ingredients to it. Here are a few variations you can try, but have fun coming up with your own combinations from whatever is in your fridge:

- Browned sausage and fresh spinach.
- Chopped bacon, sliced fresh mushrooms, and fresh spinach.
- Sliced black olives, sliced red peppers, and chopped fresh parsley.
- Diced ham, sliced green peppers, and sliced scallions.

COOKING TIP You can use a greased muffin tin with this recipe to create individual egg bites. Just make sure to evenly distribute all the ingredients among the muffin cups.

Per Batch

Calories: 1747; Total Fat: 154g; Carbs: 10g; Net Carbs: 10g; Fiber: 0g; Protein: 83g

Per Serving

Calories: 437; Total Fat: 39g; Carbs: 3g; Net Carbs: 3g; Fiber: 0g; Protein: 21g

SAUSAGE BREAKFAST STACKS

The best part about making keto-friendly breakfasts is how many simple ingredients can be combined to give you the perfect healthy fat–filled meal. Sausage patties topped with mashed avocado and a gooey, sunny-side-up egg is the perfect start to a morning.

30-MINUTE

SERVES 2

PREP 10 minutes

COOK 15 minutes

8 ounces ground pork

½ teaspoon garlic powder

½ teaspoon onion powder

2 tablespoons ghee, divided

2 large eggs

1 avocado

Pink salt

Freshly ground black pepper

1. Preheat the oven to 375°F.

2. In a medium bowl, mix well to combine the ground pork, garlic powder, and onion powder. Form the mixture into 2 patties.

3. In a medium skillet over medium-high heat, melt 1 tablespoon of ghee.

4. Add the sausage patties and cook for 2 minutes on each side, until browned.

5. Transfer the sausage to a baking sheet. Cook in the oven for 8 to 10 minutes, until cooked through.

6. Add the remaining 1 tablespoon of ghee to the skillet. When it is hot, crack the eggs into the skillet and cook without disturbing for about 3 minutes, until the whites are opaque and the yolks have set.

7. Meanwhile, in a small bowl, mash the avocado.

8. Season the eggs with pink salt and pepper.

9. Remove the cooked sausage patties from the oven.

10. Place a sausage patty on each of two warmed plates. Spread half of the mashed avocado on top of each sausage patty, and top each with a fried egg. Serve hot.

SUBSTITUTION TIP You can use precooked frozen sausage patties for an even quicker breakfast. Just make sure they are sugar-free.

Per Batch

Calories: 1066; Total Fat: 88g; Carbs: 14g; Net Carbs: 5g; Fiber: 9g; Protein: 57g

Per Serving

Calories: 533; Total Fat: 44g; Carbs: 7g; Net Carbs: 3g; Fiber: 5g; Protein: 29g